Abigail's Smile

A story about a child with EA/TEF
(Esophageal Atresia/ Tracheoesophageal Fistula)

Written By:
Ami Hays

Illustrated by:
Charlie Layton

Abigail's Smile

Copyright 2015 Ami Hays

All rights reserved under the U.S. copyright law.

ISBN-13:978-1508619208

DISCLAIMER

This book is meant to be helpful in educating families and friends of EA/TEF children. Please always consult a medical professional for advice on your child's medical condition and care.

DEDICATION

To my beautiful Abigail,
and all the EA/TEF children everywhere.

THANK YOU

To my daughter's Abigail, Carlie, and Siobhan who inspired me to write this book. I love you.

To my husband, who is a phenomenal Daddy and has supported me with this book from the moment I wanted to do it.

To my parents, who have taught me strength in pain and were the first ears to hear this book and see my vision with wanting to do it.

To the illustrator, Charlie Layton, who made this book come alive with his talent, time, and heartfelt contribution. This book could not have been possible without Charlie.

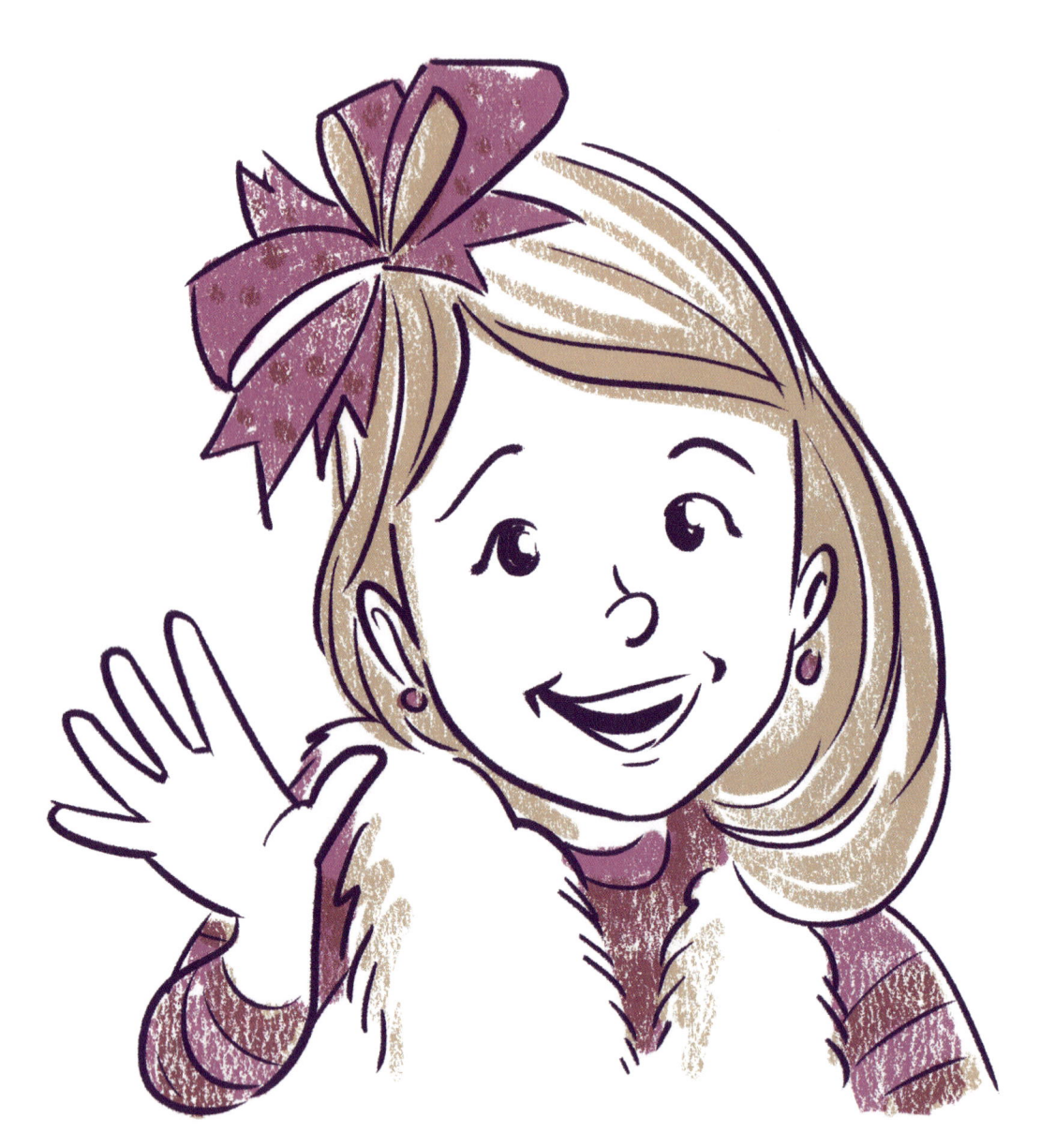

Hi, I am Abigail!

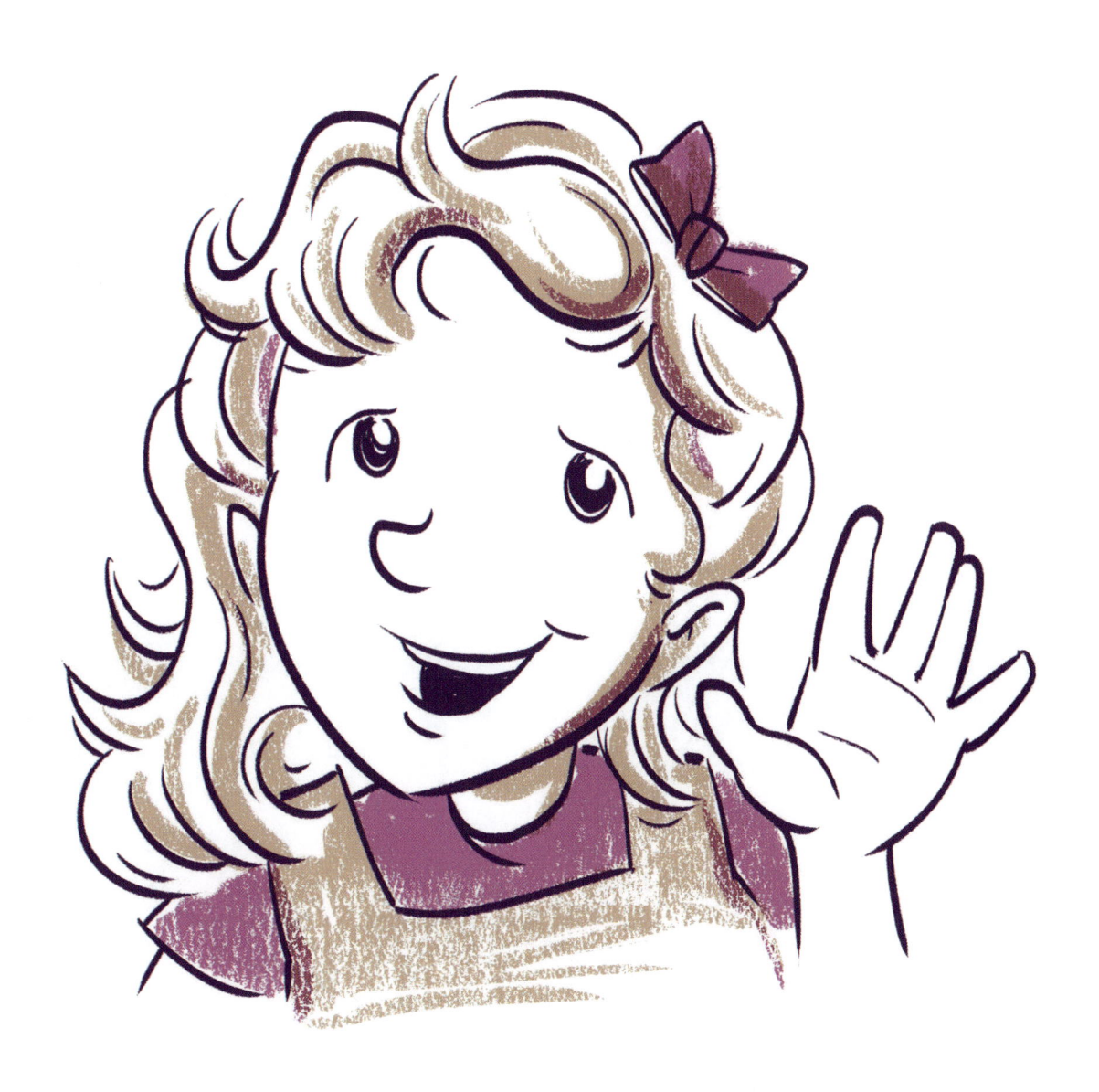

This is my little sister Carlie.

We are both very much the same, yet we are both very much different.

I am small,

Carlie is tall.

I have straight brown hair.

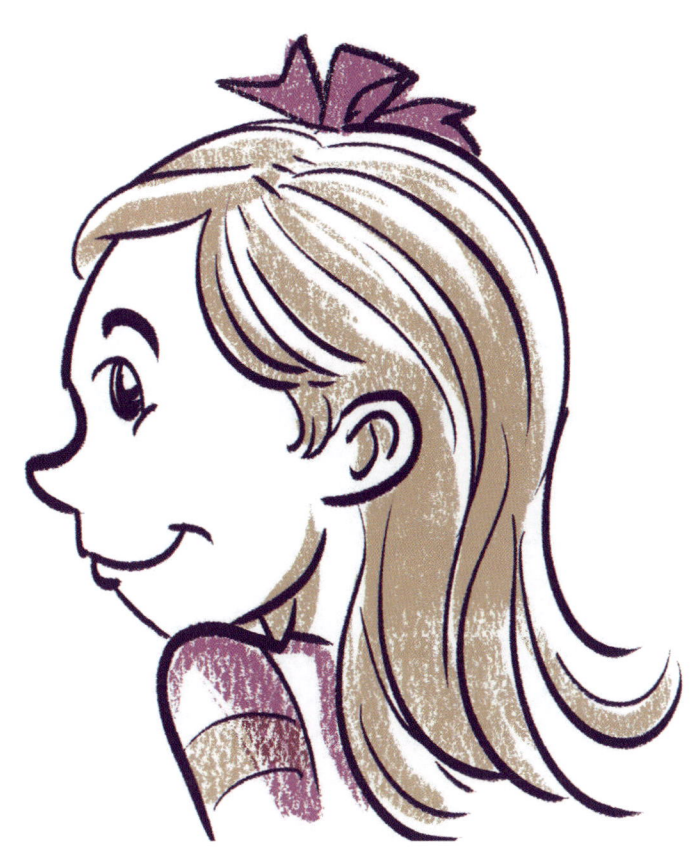

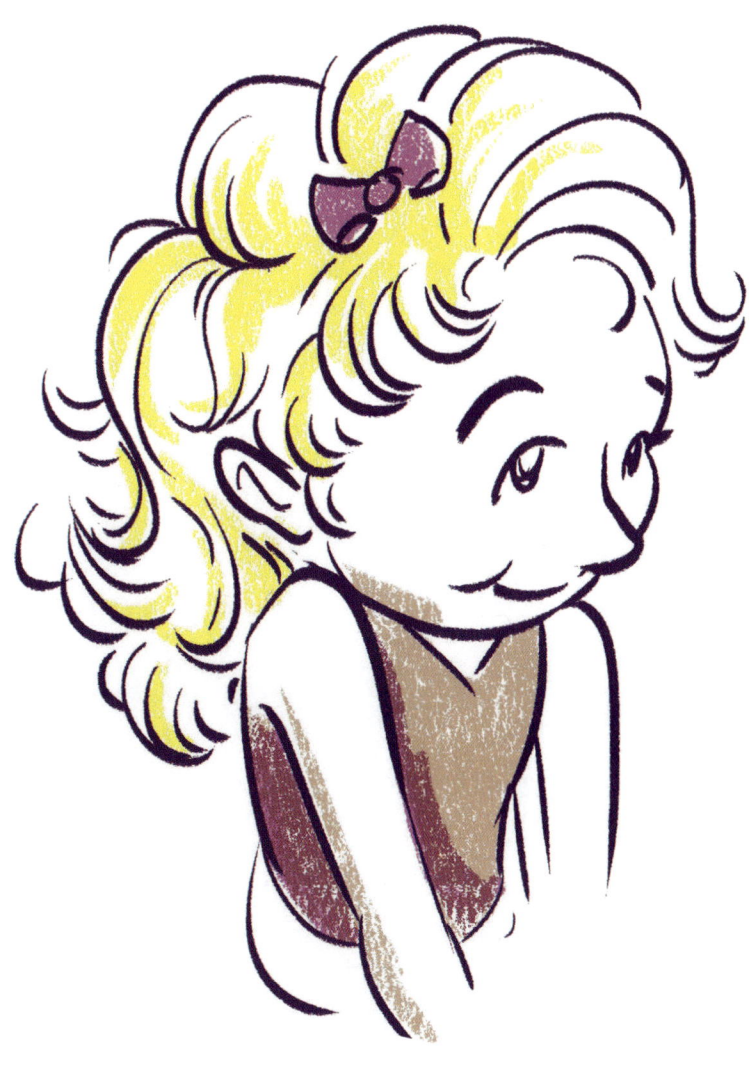

Carlie has curly blonde hair.

My eyes are the color green.
Carlie's are the color blue.

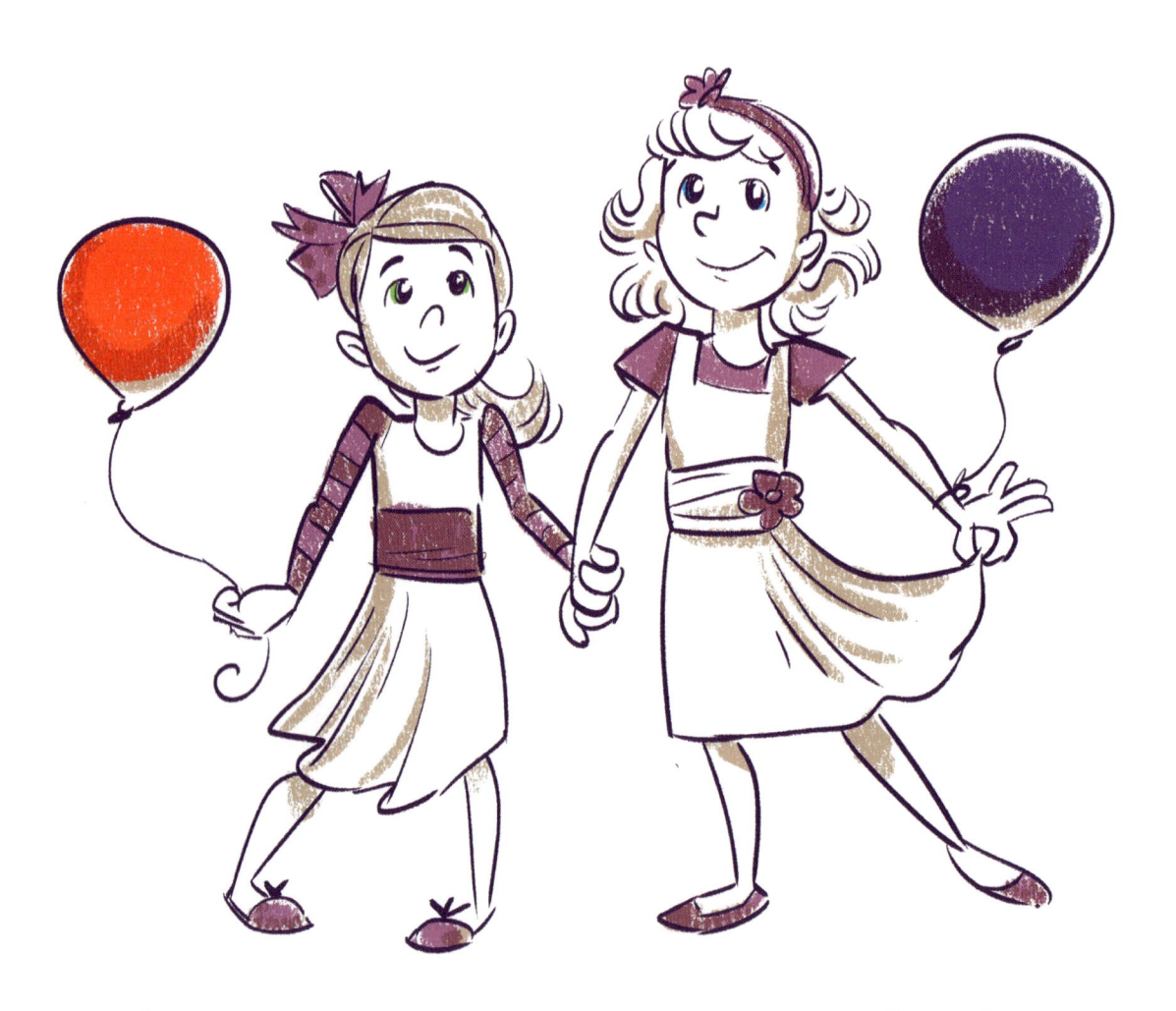

I like the color red and Carlie likes
the color purple.

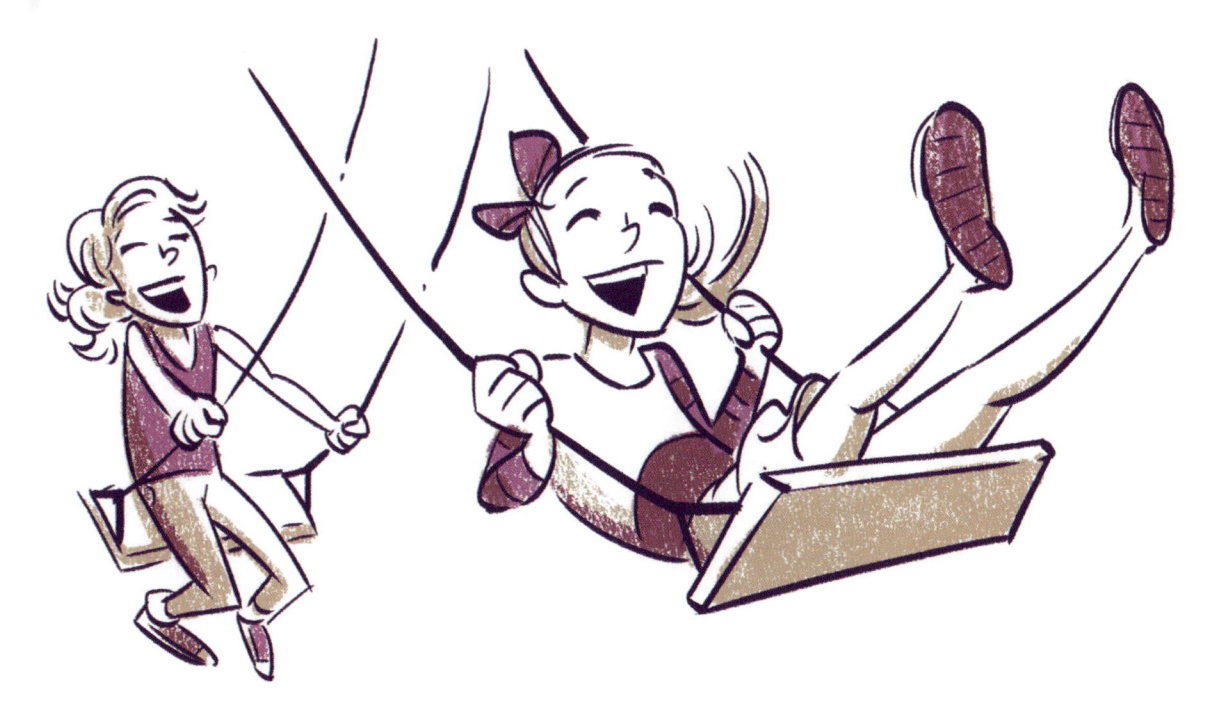

We both like to play on our swing set and in our sandbox.

We can both put our shoes on and we can both take our shoes off.

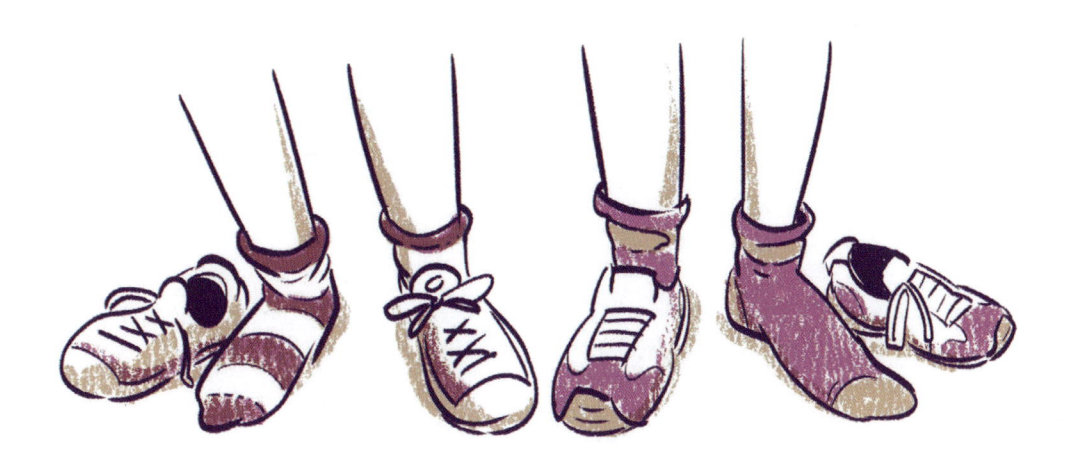

Carlie and I are very different on the inside.

We both have an esophagus, (e-soph-a-gus) or as I call it my throat.

Our throats help us swallow our food from our mouth to our stomach.

Carlie and my throat's look and act different.

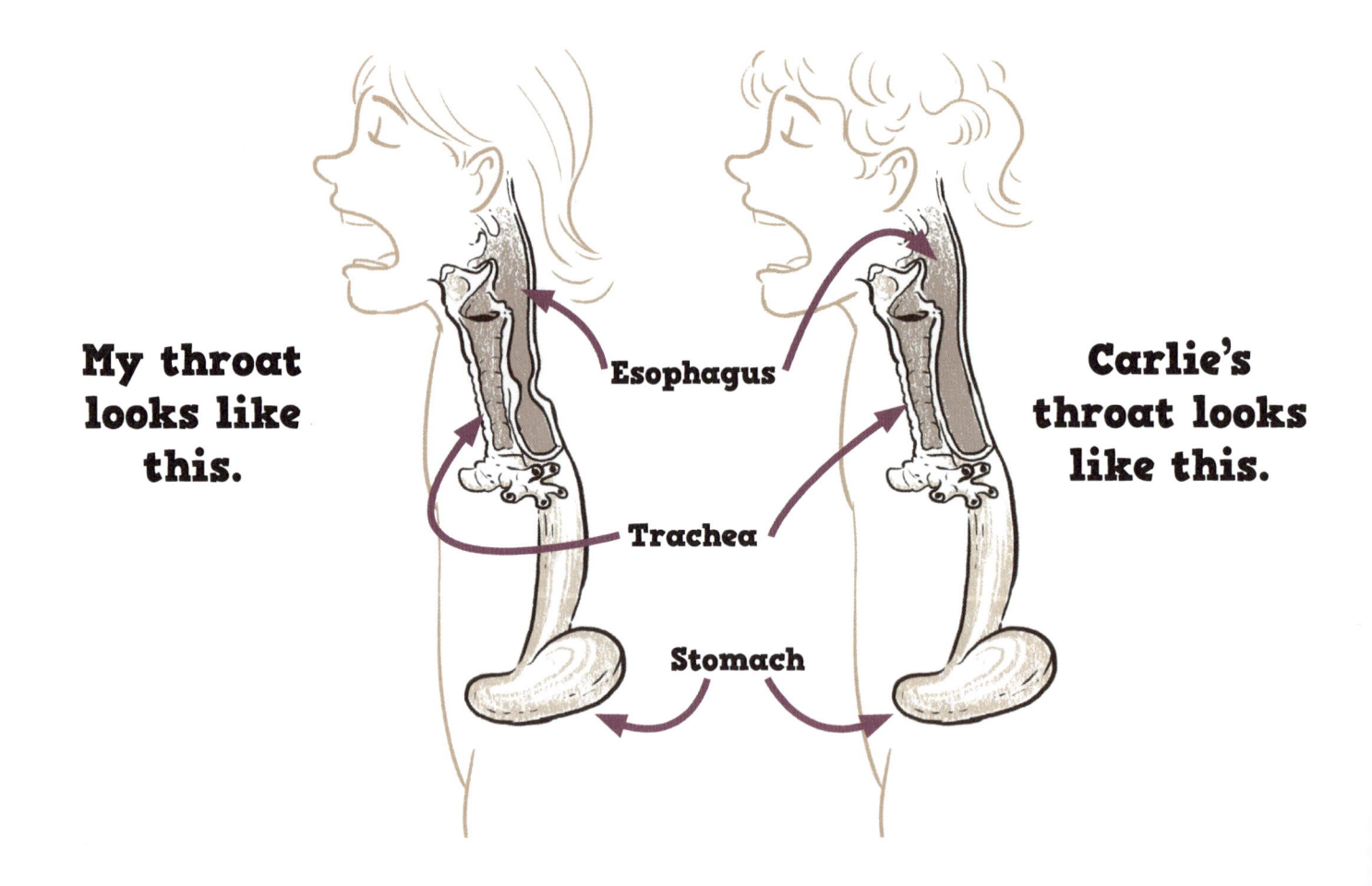

My throat looks like this.

Esophagus

Trachea

Stomach

Carlie's throat looks like this.

**We both like to eat,
but sometimes I have to eat different foods.**

**Food goes down my throat
different than Carlie's.**

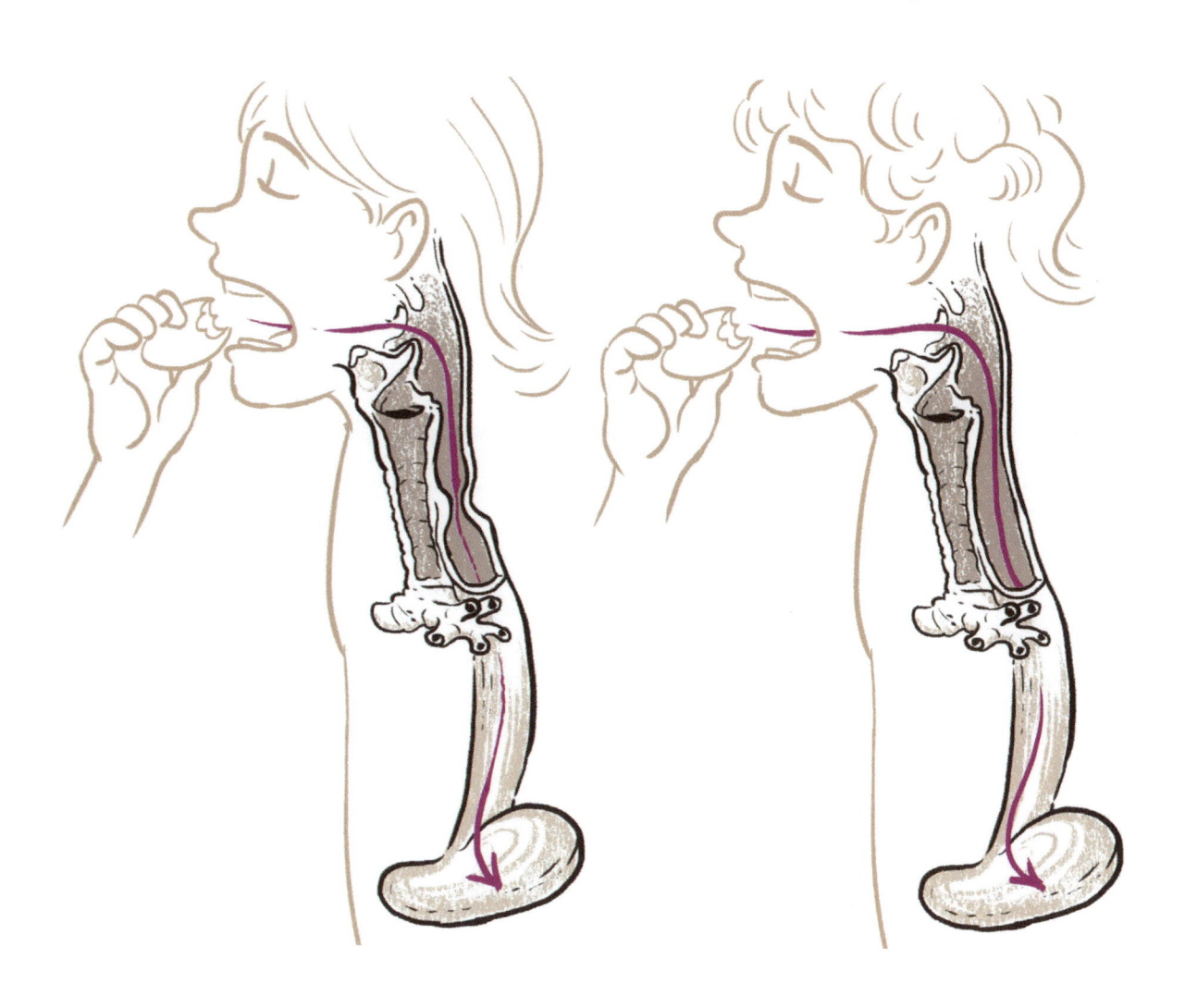

Sometimes food hurts my throat when I swallow.

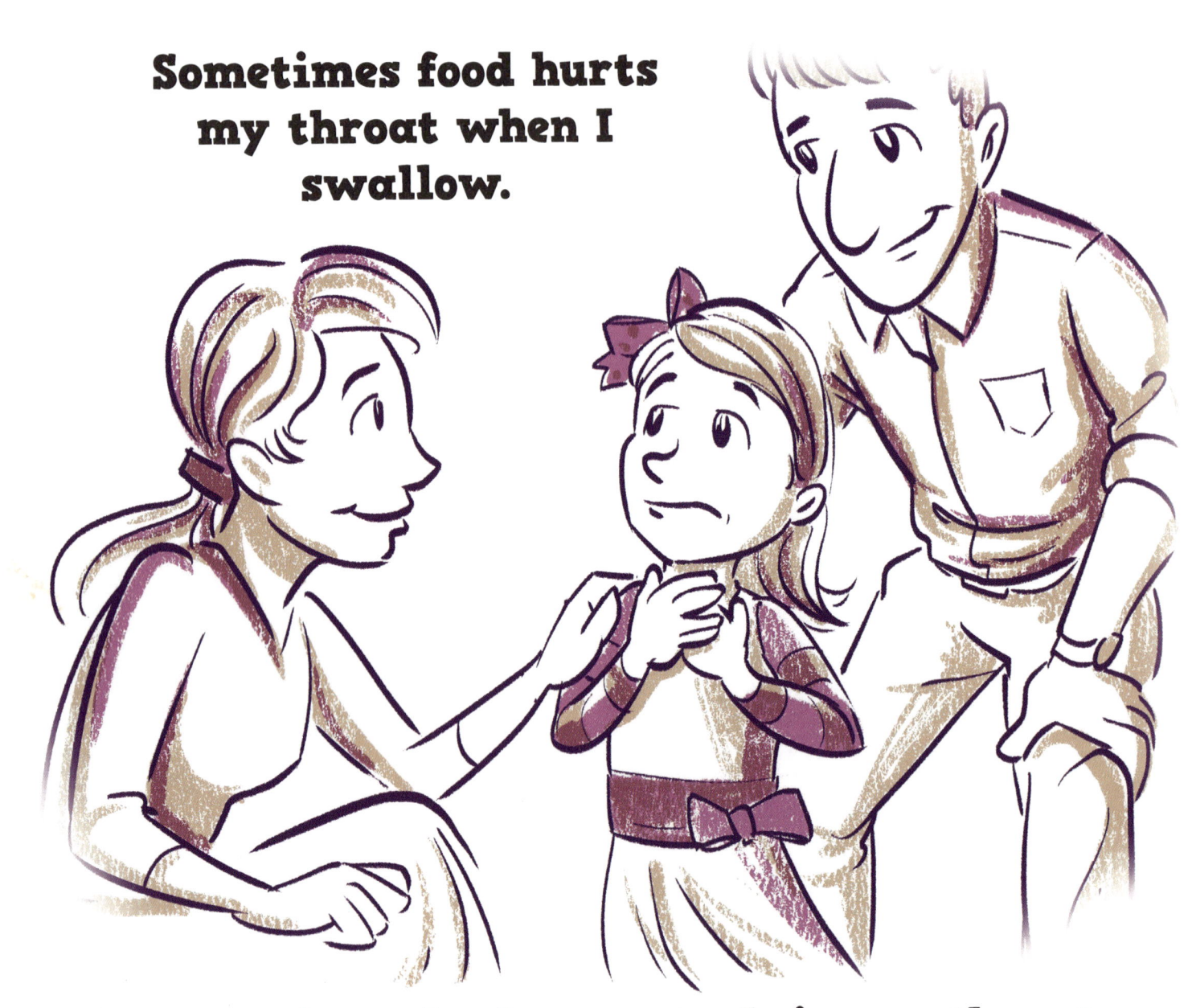

Or sometimes food gets stuck in my throat. My Mommy and Daddy help me.

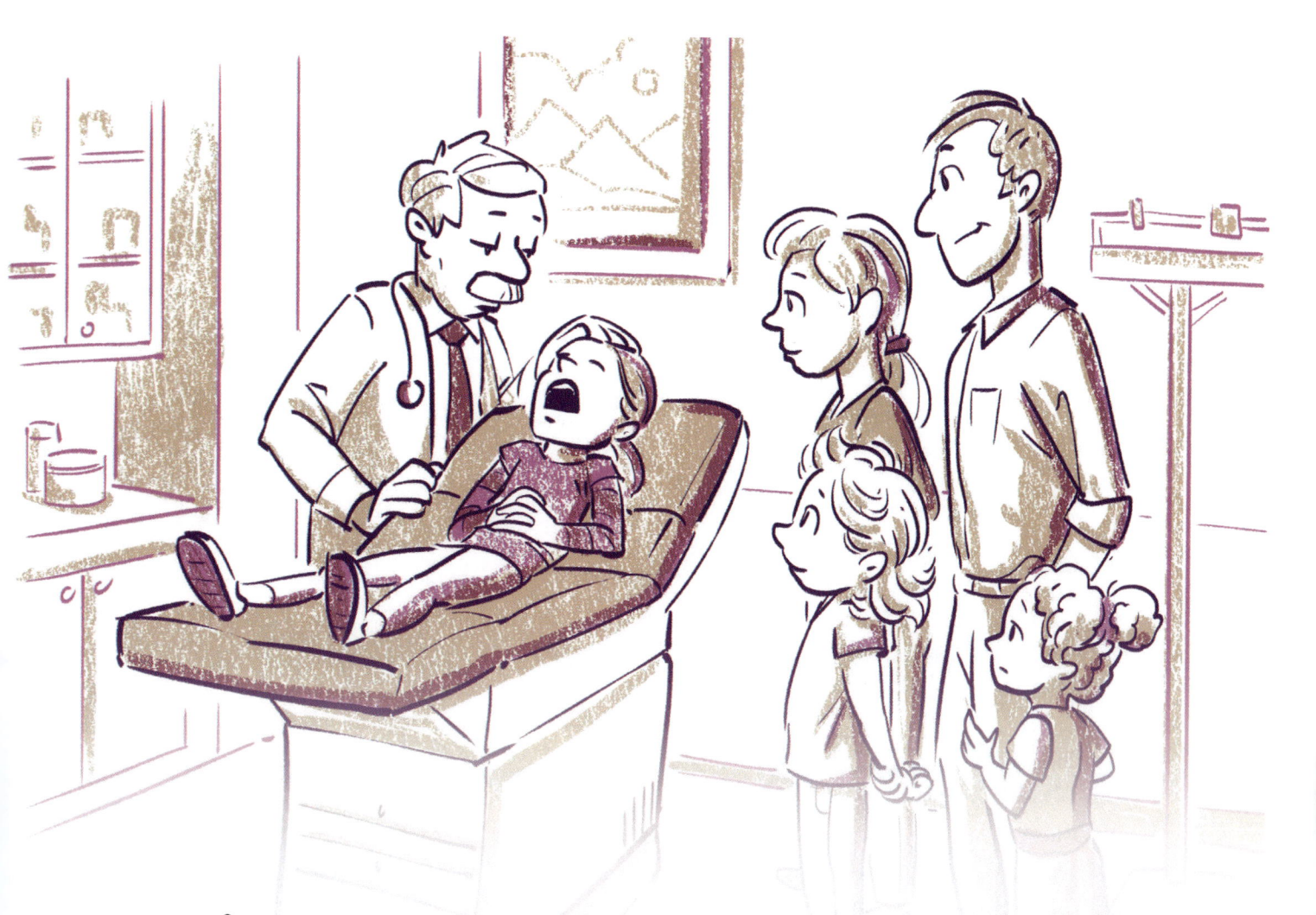

I might cry or feel a little scared when this happens.

My Mommy and Daddy say it is okay.
I go to my doctor.

He looks at my throat and keeps me safe.

The doctor says I can not eat certain foods such as:
hotdogs, steak, grapes, hard or sticky candies, and a few other things.

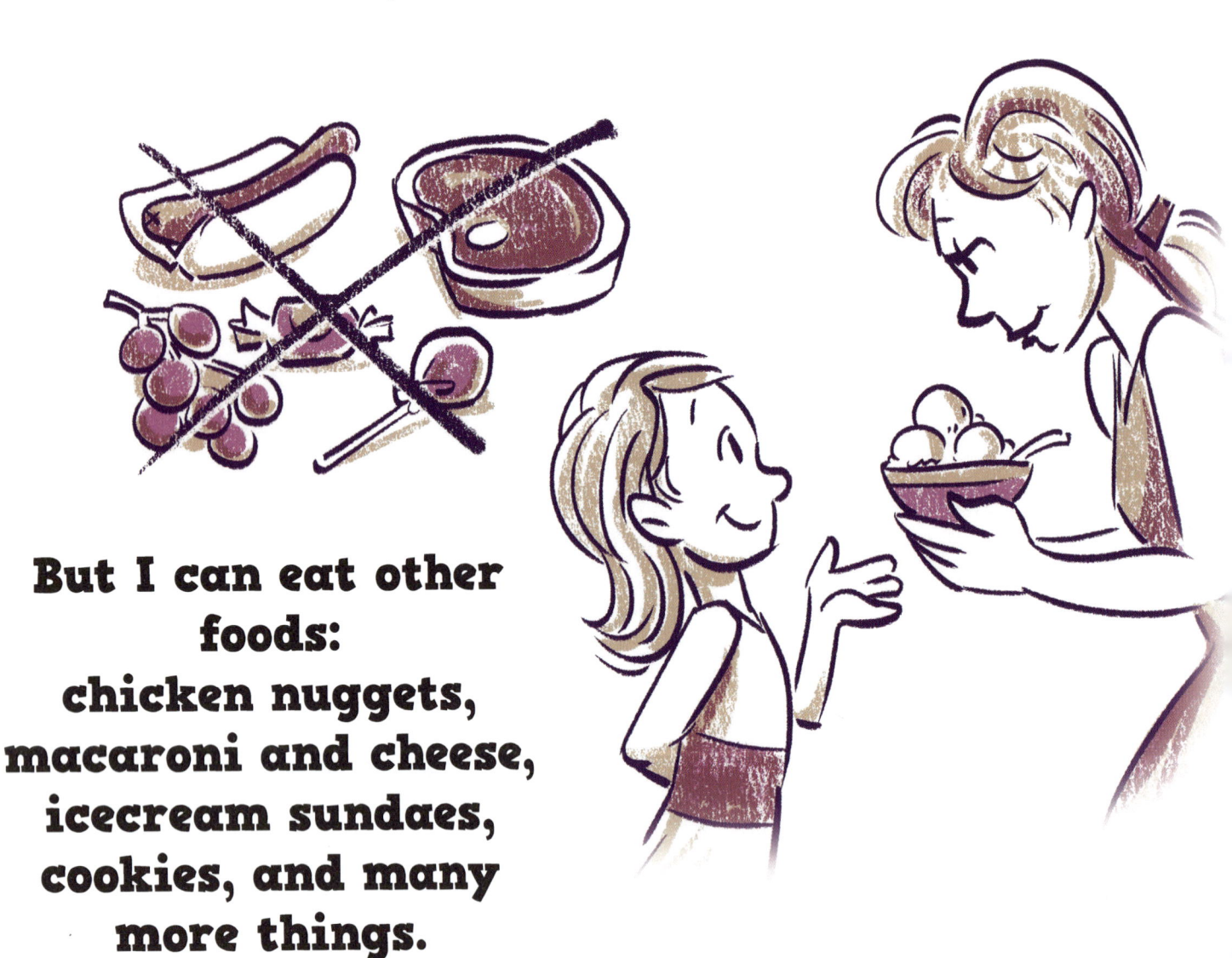

But I can eat other foods:
chicken nuggets, macaroni and cheese, icecream sundaes, cookies, and many more things.

My esophagus makes me a little different than my sister and my friends.

But I can still do many things they do.

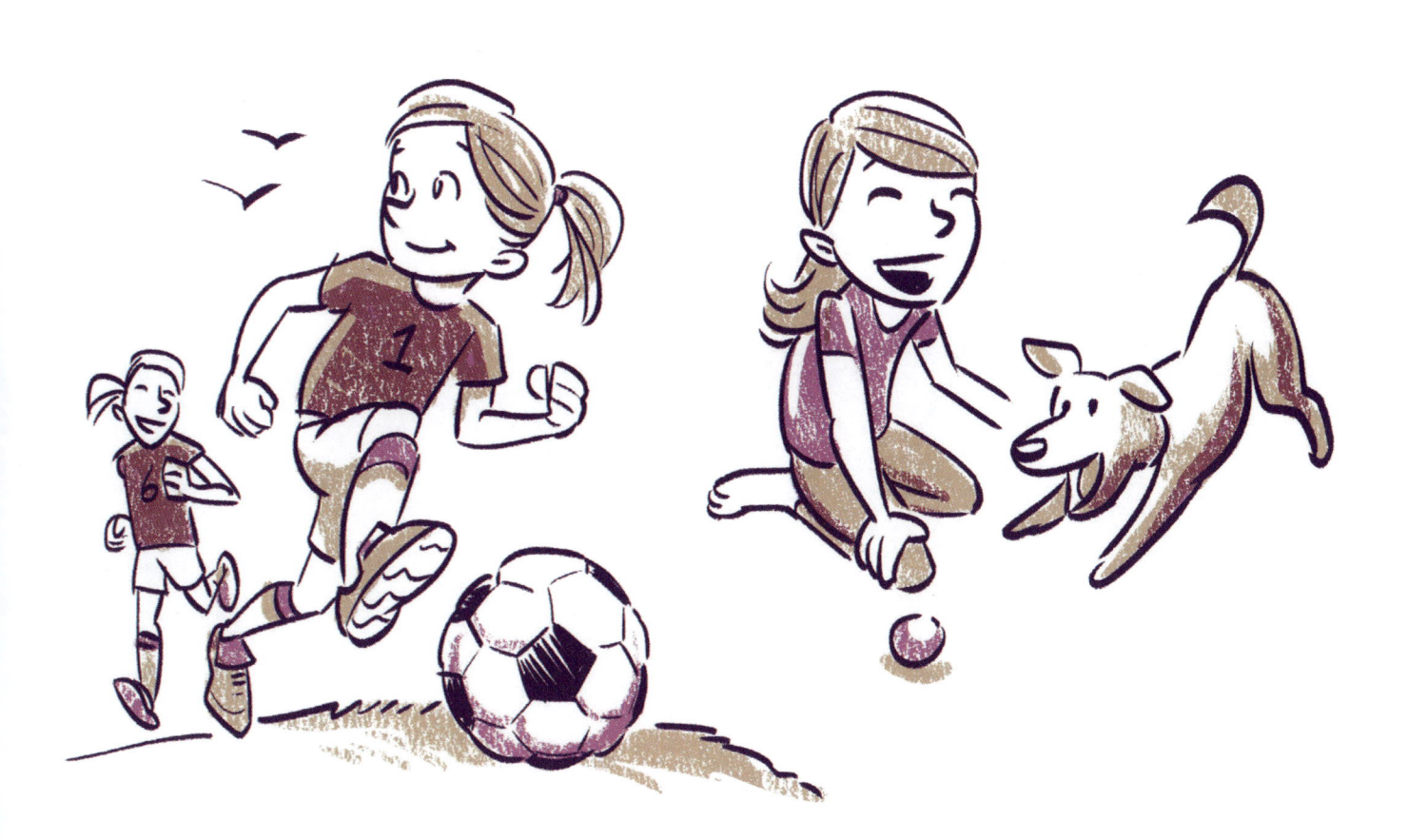

My esophagus may be different,
but I am a happy little girl.

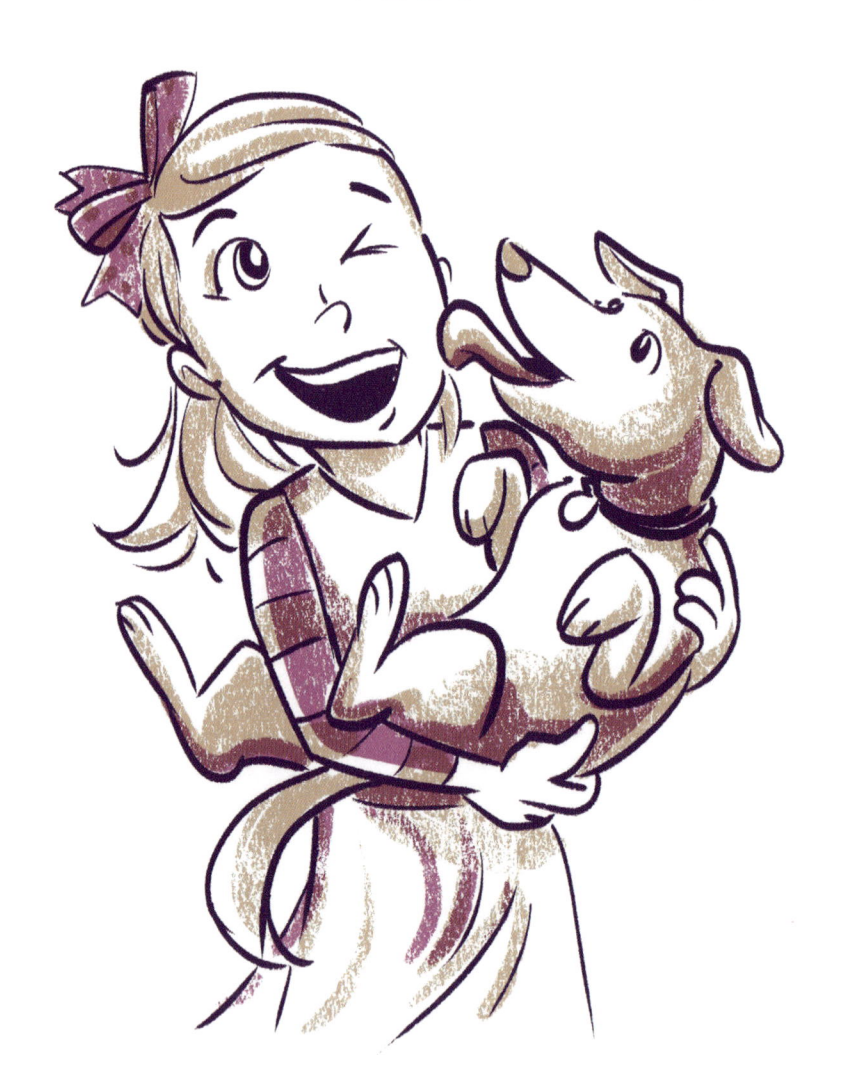

Who Loves To Smile!

Helpful Resources

MedlinePlus Encyclopedia:
Tracheoesophageal Fistula and Esophageal Atresia Repair

Boston Children's Hospital - Esophageal Atresia Treatment Program

Facebook Support Groups:
Kids born with Tracheoesophageal Fistula (TEF) & Esophageal Atresia (EA)
US: Bridging the GAP of EA/TEF
EA/TEF Family Support Connection

Glossary of terms related to EA/TEF

Esophagus:
Tube going from the throat to the stomach

Trachea (airway):
Tube going from the throat to the windpipe and lungs

Fistula:
An abnormal connection between two parts inside of the body.

Esophageal Atresia (EA):
A rare birth defect in which a baby is born without part of the esophagus (the tube that connects the mouth to the stomach). There are several types, in most cases the upper esophagus ends and does not connect with lower esophagus and stomach.

Tracheoesophageal Fistula (TEF):
A rare birth defect where an abnormal connection is between the trachea (windpipe) and esophagus. There are several types, in most cases the lower esophagus connects with the trachea (airway). Reflux from the stomach (gastric juices) can pass through the lower part of the esophagus, through the fistula, and into the lungs. The top part of the esophagus allows saliva or anything swallowed to go into the lungs.

Tracheomalacia:
Weakening or abnormal collapse of the trachea walls. This can be severe in a TEF child because the "C shaped" rings made of cartilage that help your airway stay open are not there or are damaged where the esophagus had once been abnormally connected. (This can also happen in a newborn when the cartilage in the trachea has not developed properly).

Stricture:
Narrowing of the esophagus, making it difficult to swallow, develops post surgery because scar tissue grows at the surgery site. In extreme situations a dilation will need to be performed.

Esophageal Dilation:
A procedure where the doctor dilates, or stretches, a narrowed area of the esophagus. The doctor places a tube-shaped device into the esophagus to widen the narrowed part. This procedure makes it easier to swallow.

Made in the USA
Charleston, SC
26 March 2015